GUIDE TO BECOMING VEGAN

ROBERT STJEP.

978-1-4466-5295-4
Imprint: lulu.com

This book is dedicated to all who aspire to make a change for a better, kinder, and more sustainable world. To my family, for their unwavering support and love, and to the countless individuals who inspire and drive the vegan movement forward. May this guide serve as a stepping stone on your journey towards compassion and wellness.

Welcome to "Guide to Becoming Vegan" – a journey into the heart of compassionate living. If you're holding this book, you're either curious about veganism or ready to embark on a life-altering path. This guide is designed to support, inform, and inspire you, regardless of where you are in your journey.

The decision to become vegan often stems from a blend of ethical, environmental, and health concerns. It's a choice that speaks of your commitment to a more sustainable, kinder world. However, transitioning to a vegan lifestyle is not just about changing your diet; it's about embracing a philosophy that touches every aspect of your life.

In these pages, you will find a comprehensive exploration of what it means to live vegan. From understanding the nutritional foundations to mastering vegan cooking, from navigating social situations to advocating for animal rights, this guide covers it all. We will delve into the practical aspects of vegan living, offering you tools, tips, and insights to make your transition smooth and enjoyable.

You might have questions, doubts, and perhaps some misconceptions about veganism. That's completely normal. This book aims to address these concerns, providing you with evidence-based information and real-life strategies. Whether you're a curious omnivore, a vegetarian looking to take the next step, or a new vegan seeking guidance, this guide is for you.

Remember, becoming vegan is not about perfection; it's about making choices that align more closely with your values of compassion, health, and sustainability. Every step you take on this path makes a difference. So, let's embark on this journey together – one meal, one day, one choice at a time.

Welcome to the world of vegan living.

Veganism is more than just a diet; it's a lens through which we view our relationship with the world around us. It's a commitment to living in a way that seeks to exclude, as far as is possible and practicable, all forms of exploitation of, and cruelty to, animals for food, clothing, or any other purpose. But what does this really mean in our daily lives, and why do people choose this path?

Let's start by exploring the roots of veganism. The term 'vegan' was coined in 1944 by Donald Watson, who, along with a group of vegetarians, formed the Vegan Society. They chose to avoid dairy and eggs, not just meat. Their philosophy was grounded not only in health concerns but also in a deep respect for animals. Today, veganism has grown into a global movement, encompassing a range of ethical, environmental, and health motivations.

Consider Sarah, a 30-year-old graphic designer from Portland. She became vegan after learning about the environmental impact of animal agriculture. For Sarah, every meal is a chance to reduce her carbon footprint. She represents a growing number of people who are turning to veganism out of concern for the planet. The production of animal-based products is a leading cause of greenhouse gas emissions, deforestation, and water usage. By choosing plant-based alternatives, Sarah feels empowered in her ability to make a positive impact.

Then there's Michael, a former college athlete from Atlanta, who switched to a vegan diet to improve his health. After learning about the correlation between animal products and chronic diseases, he decided to eliminate meat and dairy from his diet. Within months, he noticed significant improvements in his energy levels, recovery times, and overall health.

Michael's story is not unique; many people report similar health benefits after switching to a vegan diet.

Ethical considerations are also a central pillar of veganism. Take the case of Priya, an animal rights activist from London. For her, veganism is a stand against animal cruelty. She was moved by undercover footage from factory farms and decided she could no longer contribute to a system that treats animals as commodities. Priya's choice is a reflection of a compassionate lifestyle, extending empathy and respect to all living beings.

But veganism is not without its challenges. Common concerns include getting enough protein, iron, and other nutrients. Yet, with a well-planned diet, these concerns can be easily addressed. Plant-based sources of protein, such as lentils, beans, tofu, and quinoa, are abundant and can provide all the essential amino acids needed. Iron can be found in foods like spinach, lentils, and fortified cereals. It's important to note that vitamin B12, an essential nutrient, is not naturally present in plant foods. However, it can be easily obtained through fortified foods or supplements.

The rise of veganism has also transformed the food industry. Supermarkets and restaurants are increasingly catering to vegan diets, making it easier than ever to find plant-based options. From almond milk to vegan burgers, the variety and availability of vegan products have exploded in recent years.

But veganism is not just about what you eat. It extends to other areas of life, such as clothing, cosmetics, and entertainment. Vegans avoid leather, wool, silk, and other animal-derived materials, opting instead for alternatives like cotton, linen, and synthetic fabrics. Similarly, they choose cosmetics and household products that are not tested on animals and do not contain animal-derived ingredients.

As we continue through this book, we'll explore these aspects in greater detail, providing practical advice and tips to help you navigate the world of veganism. Whether you're motivated by health, environmental concerns, or ethical considerations, this journey is about making choices that align with your values. It's about being mindful of the impact of your actions and striving to live in harmony with the world around us.

Welcome to the enriching and rewarding path of veganism.

Embarking on a vegan journey brings with it the joy of discovering a plethora of plant-based foods, each with its unique nutritional profile. Understanding these basics is crucial to maintaining a healthy and balanced vegan diet. It's about more than just removing animal products from your meals; it's about replacing them with nutrient-rich plant-based alternatives.

The cornerstone of a nutritious vegan diet is variety. This ensures a wide range of essential nutrients, each playing a vital role in maintaining good health. Consider the rainbow of fruits and vegetables available; they're not just pleasing to the eye but packed with vitamins, minerals, and fiber. Take kale, for instance, a powerhouse of nutrients, rich in vitamins A, C, and K, calcium, and iron. Then there's quinoa, a complete protein containing all nine essential amino acids, which is also a great source of fiber and B vitamins.

A common misconception about vegan diets is the potential for protein deficiency. However, many plant-based foods are rich in protein. For example, lentils and chickpeas not only provide protein but are also excellent sources of fiber, iron, and folate. Tofu, derived from soybeans, is another versatile and protein-rich food that can be used in a variety of dishes, from stir-fries to smoothies.

Let's take a look at Emily, a software developer and a vegan food enthusiast. When she first adopted a vegan diet, she was concerned about getting enough protein. However, by incorporating a variety of plant proteins like beans, lentils, tofu, and tempeh into her meals, she not only met her protein needs but also discovered an exciting world of new flavors and textures.

Another essential aspect of a vegan diet is ensuring adequate intake of essential fatty acids, particularly omega-3s. While fish is often touted as the best source of omega-3s, flaxseeds, chia seeds, hemp seeds, and walnuts are excellent plant-based alternatives. Emily makes it a point to sprinkle ground flaxseeds on her oatmeal or add chia seeds to her smoothies to boost her omega-3 intake.

Vitamins and minerals are also key considerations. Vitamin B12, typically found in animal products, needs particular attention in a vegan diet. Fortified foods, such as plant milks, cereals, and nutritional yeast, or supplements can effectively meet this need. For instance, Emily enjoys a sprinkle of nutritional yeast on her pasta, not just for its cheesy flavor but also for its B12 content.

Iron is another nutrient that requires attention. Plant-based iron sources, like spinach, legumes, and fortified cereals, are best absorbed when combined with vitamin C-rich foods. For example, a salad of spinach, strawberries, and citrus dressing is not only delicious but also a smart way to boost iron absorption.

Calcium, essential for bone health, can be found in fortified plant milks, tofu, and leafy green vegetables. Emily makes sure to include these in her daily meals.

Additionally, exposure to sunlight helps in vitamin D synthesis, crucial for calcium absorption and overall health.

It's also important to be mindful of consuming enough calories, especially for those who are highly active. Plant-based foods tend to be less calorie-dense than animal products. This means vegans may need to eat larger quantities or choose higher-calorie foods, such as nuts and seeds, to meet their energy needs.

Lastly, hydration plays a crucial role in a vegan diet. Water, herbal teas, and other non-caffeinated beverages can keep energy levels up and support overall health. Emily makes it a habit to carry a reusable water bottle, ensuring she stays hydrated throughout the day.

In summary, a well-planned vegan diet, rich in a variety of plant-based foods, can provide all the necessary nutrients for a healthy lifestyle. By understanding these nutritional basics and incorporating a wide range of fruits, vegetables, whole grains, legumes, nuts, and seeds, vegans can enjoy a nutritious and satisfying diet. As we progress through this guide, we'll delve deeper into how to craft delicious, balanced vegan meals that cater to all your nutritional needs.

Imagine standing at the threshold of a significant life change, one that promises not only personal growth but also a positive impact on the planet and its inhabitants. This is the essence of transitioning to a vegan lifestyle, a journey that is as rewarding as it is profound. It's a path lined with discoveries, challenges, and a deepening appreciation for the power of choice.

Let's meet Alex, a high school teacher from Chicago, who decided to go vegan after watching a documentary about food and sustainability. The decision was clear, but the question of 'how' loomed large. Like many, Alex wondered how to replace his usual meals with vegan alternatives, how to handle social situations, and how to ensure he was getting the right nutrients.

The key to a successful transition is to take it one step at a time. For Alex, it started with small, manageable changes. He began by swapping out dairy milk for almond milk in his morning coffee. He found that exploring plant-based milk alternatives was not only easy but also exciting. There are so many options available – soy, oat, almond, rice, and even hemp milk, each with its unique taste and texture.

Next, Alex focused on learning to read labels. This is an essential skill for anyone embarking on a vegan journey. Many products that appear vegan at first glance may contain hidden animal-derived ingredients. Learning the names of these ingredients is crucial. For example, casein and whey, often found in bread and baked goods, are derived from milk. Gelatin, commonly used in gummy candies and desserts, is made from animal collagen. Armed with this knowledge, Alex became more confident in making vegan choices while shopping.

Another critical aspect of transitioning is finding vegan alternatives for favorite meals. Alex loved pizza, so he set out to create a vegan version. He discovered a range of plant-based cheeses and experimented with toppings like artichokes, olives, mushrooms, and bell peppers. His vegan pizza nights became a hit with his family, showing that vegan food can be just as delicious and satisfying as non-vegan options.

Meal planning also plays a vital role in a smooth transition. Alex started to plan his meals for the week, ensuring he had a variety of foods to meet his nutritional needs. He learned to cook simple vegan dishes, gradually expanding his repertoire. Websites, cookbooks, and vegan cooking channels became his go-to resources for recipes and cooking tips.

Eating out, initially a challenge, became easier with a bit of research. Alex found that many restaurants offer vegan options, and even those that don't can usually accommodate requests. He learned to communicate his dietary preferences clearly and politely, discovering that most chefs are more than willing to cater to vegan needs.

As Alex's journey progressed, he found support in the vegan community. Joining local vegan groups and online forums provided him with a sense of belonging and a wealth of shared knowledge and experiences. He also learned the importance of self-compassion. Transitioning to a vegan lifestyle is a process, and it's okay to make mistakes along the way.

In addition to dietary changes, Alex began to consider other aspects of a vegan lifestyle, such as clothing, cosmetics, and household products. He started to choose cruelty-free and vegan options, extending his commitment to compassion beyond his plate.

The transition to veganism is a deeply personal and individual journey. It's about finding what works for you, at your own pace, and enjoying the process of discovery. As Alex's story illustrates, each small step brings its own rewards and leads to a more compassionate, conscious, and sustainable way of living. In the next chapters, we will delve deeper into the practical aspects of vegan living, offering more insights and guidance to support your journey.

Imagine opening your kitchen to a new world of flavors, textures, and ingredients; a culinary adventure waiting to be embarked upon. Vegan cooking and meal planning are not just about removing animal products from your diet, but about exploring a rich tapestry of plant-based foods, each offering its unique contribution to your meals. It's an exciting journey, filled with creativity and discovery.

Let's take a journey with Jasmine, a busy marketing executive from New York City, who recently decided to adopt a vegan lifestyle. At first, the prospect of vegan cooking seemed daunting. She wondered, "What will I cook? Will it be time-consuming? Can vegan meals be both nutritious and delicious?" But as Jasmine soon discovered, with a little planning and a dash of creativity, vegan cooking can be simple, enjoyable, and incredibly satisfying.

One of the first steps in Jasmine's culinary journey was to stock her kitchen with vegan essentials. She focused on versatile ingredients that could be used in a variety of dishes. Beans, lentils, tofu, tempeh, whole grains, nuts, seeds, a wide array of fruits and vegetables, plant-based milks, and spices became the staples of her pantry. She found that having these ingredients on hand made meal preparation easier and more enjoyable. Next, Jasmine explored the art of meal planning. She started small, planning just a few days at a time, gradually building up to planning a week's worth of meals. This approach not only saved her time during the week but also helped her to ensure a varied and balanced diet. She found inspiration in vegan cookbooks and online resources, often spending Sunday afternoons preparing a few dishes that could be enjoyed throughout the week.

Breakfasts became an exciting mix of smoothie bowls topped with nuts and seeds, oatmeal with fresh fruits, or avocado toast on whole-grain bread. For lunches, Jasmine mastered the art of the Buddha bowl – a simple yet satisfying meal comprising a grain, a protein source like beans or tofu, and a variety of vegetables, all topped with a delicious dressing. Dinners were an opportunity to experiment. Jasmine discovered the versatility of tofu, using it in stir-fries, curries, and even as a base for vegan lasagna. She found that vegetables could be roasted, grilled, sautéed, or served raw in salads, offering endless possibilities. Her spice rack became her best friend, allowing her to travel the world through her cooking – from the rich curries of India to the zesty flavors of Mexican cuisine.

Snacks were not forgotten. Jasmine kept a supply of nuts, fruits, hummus with veggie sticks, and homemade granola bars, ensuring she always had healthy options on hand. She also explored vegan baking, finding joy in creating muffins, cookies, and cakes using plant-based ingredients.

Cooking at home also opened Jasmine's eyes to the impact of food choices on health and the environment. She felt empowered, knowing that her meals were not only nourishing her body but also aligning with her values of compassion and sustainability.

The beauty of vegan cooking lies in its flexibility and room for creativity. It's an ongoing journey of exploration, learning, and fun. For Jasmine, it became a cherished part of her day, a way to unwind and express herself.

In this chapter, we've journeyed with Jasmine through the basics of vegan cooking and meal planning. As you embark on your own culinary adventure, remember that each meal is an opportunity to nourish your body, delight your senses, and express your commitment to a kinder, more sustainable world. In the following chapters, we will continue to explore the diverse and delicious world of vegan cuisine, offering more tips, techniques, and recipes to inspire your journey.

Stepping into a grocery store as a new vegan can feel like entering a maze, filled with a multitude of choices and decisions. It's an entirely new landscape to navigate, but with a bit of know-how and planning, it can quickly become a delightful and empowering experience. This chapter is about transforming your shopping trips into an adventure of discovery, finding joy in the myriad of plant-based options available, and learning how to make choices that align with your vegan values. Let's follow the journey of Carlos, an architect from Miami, who recently embraced veganism. Initially overwhelmed by the prospect of shopping for vegan foods, Carlos quickly learned that with a few tips and strategies, he could navigate the grocery aisles with confidence and ease.

Carlos's first step was to familiarize himself with the layout of his local grocery store. He discovered that most of his vegan essentials could be found along the perimeter, where fresh produce, bread, and plant-based milk alternatives were located. He also explored the natural foods section, a treasure trove of vegan-friendly items like tofu, tempeh, whole grains, and legumes.

One of the most important skills Carlos developed was label reading. He learned to scrutinize ingredient lists, keeping an eye out for hidden animal-derived ingredients such as gelatin, casein, whey, and certain e-numbers. He also looked for certifications like "vegan" or "cruelty-free" to ensure the products aligned with his ethical choices.

Planning ahead was key to efficient and stress-free shopping. Carlos started to make a weekly meal plan and grocery list, ensuring he purchased only what he needed, reducing waste, and saving money. He found that some items, like dried beans and lentils, were more economical in bulk, while others, like certain fruits and vegetables, were best bought fresh and in smaller quantities.

Carlos also discovered the joy of exploring new foods. He experimented with different plant-based milk alternatives, from almond to oat to rice milk, each adding its unique flavor to his morning cereal or coffee. He tried a variety of meat alternatives, from seitan to textured vegetable protein, finding which ones he liked best for different types of dishes.

Seasonal produce became a new passion for Carlos. He learned that eating seasonally not only offered better flavor and nutritional value but also supported local farmers and reduced his carbon footprint. He enjoyed the challenge of creating meals based on what was in season, finding inspiration in the vibrant colors and textures of seasonal fruits and vegetables.

Carlos also explored the world of spices and herbs, understanding that these were essential in adding depth and richness to vegan dishes. He stocked his pantry with a variety of spices, learning how to use them to bring out the best in his cooking.

In addition, Carlos learned to navigate the challenges of non-food items. He started to choose household products and personal care items that were not tested on animals and were free from animal-derived ingredients. This extended his vegan principles beyond his plate and into all aspects of his lifestyle.

Over time, shopping as a vegan became second nature to Carlos. He found pleasure in the process, knowing that each choice he made was a reflection of his commitment to a healthier, more ethical, and sustainable way of living.

As we close this chapter, remember that vegan shopping is an integral part of the journey. It's about making informed choices, exploring new foods, and enjoying the process of aligning your purchases with your values. In the next chapter, we'll delve into the world of vegan recipes, offering you a collection of delicious and easy-to-make dishes to add to your culinary repertoire.

The heart of a vegan lifestyle beats in the kitchen, where the magic of transforming simple plant-based ingredients into extraordinary meals happens. This chapter is a celebration of vegan recipes – a showcase of how diverse, flavorful, and satisfying vegan food can be. Whether you are a seasoned cook or new to the kitchen, these recipes will inspire you, tantalize your taste buds, and perhaps even surprise you with the versatility and richness of vegan cuisine.

Let's join Naomi, a freelance writer and mother of two from Seattle, in her culinary adventures. Naomi, a recent convert to veganism, was initially concerned about missing her favorite dishes. However, she soon discovered that almost any dish could be "veganized" and that the process was not just simple but also incredibly fun.

One of Naomi's first forays into vegan cooking was breakfast, a meal often dominated by eggs and dairy. She started experimenting with tofu scramble, a dish that quickly became a weekend staple in her household. By crumbling firm tofu and adding turmeric, nutritional yeast, and a mix of her favorite vegetables like spinach, bell peppers, and mushrooms, she created a delicious, nutritious alternative to scrambled eggs.

For lunches, Naomi explored the world of soups and salads. She found that lentil soup, packed with vegetables and flavored with cumin and coriander, was not only hearty and warming but also rich in protein and fiber. Her salads became more adventurous, combining grains like quinoa or farro with an array of vegetables, toasted nuts, and a tangy dressing, perfect for a quick yet satisfying midday meal.

Dinners were an opportunity for Naomi to get creative. She loved Italian cuisine and learned to make vegan versions of her favorites. Her vegan lasagna, layered with cashew ricotta, spinach, and marinara sauce, was a hit with her family. She also mastered the art of making vegan pizza, topping her homemade crust with tomato sauce, vegan cheese, and a variety of vegetables like artichokes, olives, and sun-dried tomatoes.

Naomi also discovered the joy of vegan baking. She experimented with flax eggs (a mixture of ground flaxseeds and water) as an egg substitute in her baking, which worked wonderfully in cakes, muffins, and cookies. Her chocolate avocado cake became a much-requested dessert, rich, moist, and entirely plant-based.

One of Naomi's favorite recipes was a simple yet flavorful chickpea curry. She sautéed onions, garlic, and ginger, added spices like garam masala and turmeric, then cooked the chickpeas in a tomato-based sauce, finishing it with a splash of coconut milk for creaminess. Served with rice or naan, it was a comforting and satisfying meal, easy enough for a weeknight dinner.

Snacks and small bites were also part of Naomi's repertoire. She often made hummus from scratch, experimenting with different flavors like roasted red pepper or lemon and garlic. Paired with vegetable sticks or whole-grain pita, it was a healthy and delicious snack. She also enjoyed making energy balls with dates, nuts, and oats, perfect for a quick energy boost during her busy day.

Through her journey in vegan cooking, Naomi not only expanded her culinary skills but also found a new appreciation for the diversity of plant-based foods. She realized that vegan cooking is not about deprivation but about exploring new flavors and textures, about nourishing the body and soul with wholesome, compassionate choices.

In this chapter, we've shared a glimpse into the world of vegan recipes through Naomi's story. As we move forward, we invite you to continue exploring, experimenting, and enjoying the rich tapestry of vegan cuisine. The possibilities are endless, and each meal is an opportunity to celebrate the joys of plant-based eating. In the next chapter, we will dive into the intricacies of vegan nutrition, ensuring that your vegan journey is not only delicious but also nutritionally sound.

Veganism isn't just a solitary pursuit; it's a lifestyle that weaves through the social fabric of our lives. Dining out and attending social gatherings as a vegan can initially seem daunting. Yet, with a touch of planning and communication, these experiences can be both enjoyable and an opportunity to showcase the richness of vegan cuisine to others. This chapter delves into the nuances of maintaining a vegan lifestyle while navigating the diverse terrains of restaurants, family dinners, and social events.

Let's join Oliver, a graphic designer and music enthusiast from Austin, who recently embraced veganism. He loved dining out and attending social gatherings but was initially apprehensive about how his new lifestyle choice would fit into these scenarios. Oliver's journey is a testament to how one can gracefully and joyfully integrate veganism into their social life.

Oliver's first challenge was eating out. He started by researching restaurants in his area, pleasantly surprised to find a variety of vegan or vegan-friendly options. He discovered that many restaurants, even those not specifically vegan, were willing to accommodate his dietary preferences. He made a habit of calling ahead or checking menus online to identify vegan options or dishes that could be modified.

One of his favorite finds was a Mediterranean restaurant that offered an array of vegan dishes, from hummus and falafel to stuffed grape leaves and tabbouleh. He also found that many Asian restaurants, particularly Thai and Indian, had a variety of vegan choices, thanks to their use of tofu, vegetables, and legumes, cooked in rich, flavorful sauces.

When options seemed limited, Oliver learned to be creative with the menu. He often combined side dishes to create a meal or asked the chef to omit or substitute non-vegan ingredients in a dish. He was usually met with understanding and willingness to accommodate his requests.

Social gatherings, such as family dinners and parties with friends, posed a different set of challenges. Oliver started by always offering to bring a dish to share, ensuring there would be something vegan for him to enjoy. This also became an opportunity to introduce his friends and family to vegan cuisine. His lentil walnut loaf and vegan spinach artichoke dip became crowd favorites, often requested even by his non-vegan friends.

At family dinners, Oliver communicated his dietary choices clearly and respectfully to his family. He offered to help with meal planning or cooking, making it easier for his family to accommodate his vegan diet. Over time, his family became more open and curious about veganism, often incorporating vegan dishes into their gatherings.

Potlucks were another opportunity for Oliver to showcase vegan cuisine. He found joy in preparing dishes that were not only delicious but also visually appealing. His colorful quinoa salad, dressed in a tangy lemon vinaigrette and loaded with crisp vegetables, became a staple at these events. For Oliver, attending events like weddings or company dinners required a bit of planning. He made it a habit to inform the host or event organizer of his dietary preferences well in advance. Most were accommodating, ensuring that a vegan option was available for him.

Through his experiences, Oliver learned that communication and a positive attitude were key. He approached each situation with the mindset of flexibility and understanding, finding that most people were receptive and accommodating once they understood his dietary choices.

This chapter has followed Oliver's journey, highlighting that being vegan doesn't mean sacrificing social interactions or the joy of dining out. It's about finding balance, being prepared, and embracing the opportunity to share the beauty of veganism with others. As you navigate your own social experiences as a vegan, remember that each interaction is an opportunity to positively influence others and enjoy the rich tapestry of social dining. In the next chapter, we'll explore the specific nutritional needs of different groups within the vegan community, ensuring that everyone from athletes to seniors can thrive on a vegan diet.

Embarking on a vegan lifestyle is an inclusive journey, catering to individuals from all walks of life. Each person brings unique nutritional needs based on their age, activity level, health status, and life stage. Understanding how to meet these specific needs is crucial for a wholesome and sustainable vegan lifestyle. This chapter delves into the nuances of tailoring the vegan diet to suit various groups, from athletes and children to pregnant women and seniors, ensuring everyone can thrive on a plant-based diet.

Let's start with athletes, who have higher energy and protein requirements. Meet Clara, a triathlete from San Diego, who transitioned to a vegan diet to improve her performance and recovery. Clara focuses on consuming adequate calories, primarily from carbohydrate-rich foods like whole grains, fruits, and vegetables, to fuel her rigorous training sessions. She includes protein-rich foods like tofu, lentils, quinoa, and tempeh in her meals to support muscle repair and growth. Clara also pays attention to micronutrients like iron, calcium, and vitamin B12, supplementing as necessary to meet her heightened nutritional demands. For children and teenagers, a well-planned vegan diet can provide all the necessary nutrients for growth and development. Consider the case of the Lee family from Toronto, who raised their children on a vegan diet. They ensure their children's nutritional needs are met by including a variety of fruits, vegetables, whole grains, legumes, nuts, and seeds in their meals. They pay special attention to nutrients like calcium, vitamin D, and omega-3 fatty acids, critical for growing bodies. The Lee children also take a vitamin B12 supplement, an essential practice in a vegan diet.

Pregnant and breastfeeding women have increased nutritional requirements to support the growth and development of their babies. Take Maya, a software engineer from Boston, who maintained her vegan diet throughout her pregnancy and breastfeeding period. She focuses on consuming a variety of nutrient-dense foods to meet her increased needs for protein, iron, folate, calcium, and omega-3 fatty acids. Maya consults with her healthcare provider to monitor her nutritional status and takes prenatal vitamins, including B12 and DHA (an essential omega-3 fatty acid), to ensure both she and her baby are getting all the necessary nutrients.

Seniors can also thrive on a vegan diet, although they may have specific nutritional concerns. Consider Mr. and Mrs. Patel, a retired couple living in London, who adopted a vegan diet later in life. They focus on nutrient-dense foods that are easy to chew and digest, such as cooked vegetables, soft legumes, and smoothies. They ensure adequate protein intake to maintain muscle mass and pay attention to vitamin B12, vitamin D, and calcium, which are crucial for bone health and overall well-being in older age.

Individuals with specific health conditions can also benefit from a vegan diet, provided it's well-planned and tailored to their needs. Emily, a graphic designer from Melbourne with type 2 diabetes, adopted a vegan diet to better manage her condition. She focuses on low-glycemic foods, such as leafy greens, whole grains, legumes, and nuts, to maintain stable blood sugar levels. She also includes foods rich in fiber, which helps with blood sugar control and overall digestive health.

In summary, a vegan diet can be adapted to meet the diverse needs of individuals across different life stages and physical conditions. It requires a thoughtful approach to food choices and, in some cases, supplementation. By focusing on a variety of nutrient-dense foods and consulting with healthcare professionals as needed, individuals with specific dietary needs can not only sustain but also flourish on a vegan diet.

In the next chapters, we will continue our exploration of the vegan lifestyle, addressing common challenges and misconceptions, and offering guidance to help you navigate your vegan journey with confidence and joy.

Every journey has its hurdles, and the path to veganism is no exception. Whether it's dealing with practical challenges or facing skepticism and criticism from others, navigating these obstacles is an integral part of the vegan experience. This chapter focuses on the common challenges vegans face and offers strategies for handling them with grace and resilience.

Let's take a look at the experience of David, a software engineer from Atlanta, who faced various challenges when he first adopted a vegan lifestyle. One of the initial hurdles was learning how to cook vegan meals. David, who had limited cooking experience, initially found it overwhelming to prepare different meals. He started with simple recipes, using online tutorials and vegan cooking apps. Gradually, his skills improved, and he became more confident in the kitchen, discovering that vegan cooking can be both easy and enjoyable.

Another challenge David encountered was navigating social situations, particularly family gatherings where vegan options were limited. He learned to communicate his dietary choices to his family in advance and often brought his own dishes to share. This not only ensured that he had something to eat but also gave him an opportunity to introduce his family to tasty vegan food. Over time, his family became more accommodating and even started incorporating vegan dishes into their meals.

David also faced skepticism and criticism about his diet, both in his personal and professional circles. Some questioned the nutritional adequacy of his diet, while others joked about his food choices. David equipped himself with knowledge, reading up on vegan nutrition and the benefits of a plant-based diet. This allowed him to address concerns and questions confidently and factually. He also learned to navigate these conversations with a sense of humor and patience, realizing that not everyone would understand or accept his choices. Eating out posed another challenge. While more and more restaurants are offering vegan options, there were still times when David found it difficult to find suitable meals, especially when traveling. He learned to do research ahead of time, looking up vegan-friendly restaurants or menu options. In situations where options were limited, he wasn't shy about asking for customizations to existing dishes. Most chefs and restaurants were accommodating and happy to tweak their dishes to make them vegan.

David also faced challenges related to nutrition. Ensuring a balanced intake of all essential nutrients required some learning and planning. He started using a food tracking app to monitor his nutrient intake and made sure to include a variety of foods in his diet. For nutrients that are harder to obtain from a vegan diet, like vitamin B12 and omega-3 fatty acids, he took supplements as recommended by his healthcare provider.

Through his journey, David learned that being a vegan wasn't just about what he ate; it extended to other lifestyle choices, such as clothing, cosmetics, and entertainment. He became more conscious of his purchasing decisions, choosing products that were cruelty-free and environmentally friendly.

David's experience illustrates that while the vegan journey can have its challenges, they are surmountable with the right approach and mindset. It's about being prepared, staying informed, and maintaining a positive and flexible attitude.

In this chapter, we've explored the common challenges vegans face and how to navigate them effectively. In the following chapters, we will delve deeper into the broader implications of veganism beyond diet, including its impact on the environment and animal welfare, and how to engage in advocacy and community building as part of the vegan journey.

Embarking on a vegan journey extends far beyond the boundaries of the plate. It encompasses a holistic approach to living, influencing choices in clothing, personal care, entertainment, and more. This chapter delves into the comprehensive vegan lifestyle, exploring how vegan principles can be applied in various aspects of life, illustrating that veganism is not just a diet but a way of life that reflects compassion and sustainability in every choice.

Let's consider the story of Lisa, a school teacher from Portland, who decided to embrace veganism not only in her diet but in all facets of her life. Lisa's journey into the broader aspects of veganism began with her wardrobe. She started by phasing out clothing made from animal-derived materials such as leather, wool, silk, and fur. Instead, she opted for alternatives made from cotton, linen, synthetic materials, and other cruelty-free fabrics.

This shift wasn't just about avoiding animal products; it was a stand against the industries that exploit animals for fashion. Next, Lisa turned her attention to her beauty routine. She began scrutinizing the labels of her cosmetics, skincare, and hair care products, looking for ingredients of animal origin and ensuring they were cruelty-free - not tested on animals. She found numerous brands that aligned with her vegan values, offering high-quality, ethical products. Lisa discovered that these choices not only felt right ethically but often led to products that were gentler and more natural.

In her home, Lisa made similar changes. She replaced household cleaners, detergents, and other everyday items with vegan-friendly alternatives. She learned that many common household products contain animal-derived ingredients or are tested on animals, something she was keen to avoid. She started using products made with plant-based ingredients, which were not only cruelty-free but also environmentally friendly.

Entertainment was another area where Lisa applied her vegan principles. She became more mindful of the activities she supported, choosing to avoid zoos, circuses, aquariums, and other forms of entertainment that exploit animals. Instead, she sought out animal-friendly activities like visiting animal sanctuaries, wildlife reserves, and botanical gardens, places where animals are respected and live in more natural settings.

Lisa also explored the vegan community in her city, attending meetups, potlucks, and festivals. This not only provided her with a sense of belonging but also opened up opportunities to learn from others who were walking the same path. She found support, inspiration, and friendship in these communities, which helped strengthen her commitment to veganism.

Finally, Lisa's journey extended into her professional life. As a teacher, she found ways to incorporate lessons about compassion, sustainability, and environmental stewardship into her curriculum. She encouraged her students to think critically about their food choices and the impact of these choices on the planet and its inhabitants.

Lisa's story is a testament to the fact that veganism is more than just a dietary choice; it is a comprehensive lifestyle. It reflects a commitment to making ethical, sustainable choices in every aspect of life.

This chapter has highlighted how the principles of veganism can be applied beyond diet, influencing clothing, personal care, household items, entertainment, and even professional life. In the next chapters, we will explore the environmental and ethical dimensions of veganism, deepening our understanding of how this lifestyle contributes to a more sustainable and compassionate world.

Veganism is not only a personal health choice but also a profound environmental stance. As we become more aware of our planet's fragility, understanding the environmental impact of our food choices becomes increasingly crucial. This chapter explores the connection between veganism and environmental stewardship, illustrating how adopting a plant-based lifestyle can be a powerful tool in the fight against climate change, deforestation, water scarcity, and biodiversity loss.

Meet Daniel, an environmental scientist from Boulder, Colorado, whose journey into veganism was primarily motivated by his concern for the planet. Through his research, Daniel realized the significant impact of animal agriculture on the environment. He learned that livestock farming is one of the largest contributors to greenhouse gas emissions, more than the entire transportation sector combined. This was a pivotal moment for Daniel, leading him to adopt a vegan diet as a tangible way to reduce his carbon footprint.

Daniel also discovered the immense water usage involved in animal agriculture. Producing a single pound of beef requires thousands of gallons of water, much more than plant-based foods. By choosing vegan options, he was contributing to water conservation efforts, an essential consideration in today's world where water scarcity is a growing concern.

Another environmental concern that influenced Daniel's shift to veganism was deforestation. Vast areas of forests are cleared to create grazing land for livestock or to grow crops to feed animals raised for food. This deforestation not only contributes to climate change but also leads to the loss of biodiversity. By opting for plant-based foods, Daniel was taking a stand against this destructive practice, supporting more sustainable land use.

Furthermore, Daniel was alarmed by the impact of animal agriculture on ocean health. Overfishing, along with pollution from fish farms, has led to the depletion of fish populations and damage to marine ecosystems. By eliminating fish and seafood from his diet, he was contributing to the preservation of ocean life.

Inspired by his findings, Daniel became an advocate for environmental sustainability through veganism. He started giving talks at local schools and community centers, sharing his knowledge about the environmental benefits of a plant-based diet. He emphasized that every meal is an opportunity to make a choice that benefits the planet.

Daniel's advocacy extended to his personal life as well. He started growing his own vegetables and herbs, reducing his reliance on commercially grown produce and further minimizing his environmental impact. He also supported local farmers' markets, choosing organic and locally grown produce whenever possible.

Through his journey, Daniel demonstrated that veganism is a powerful way to live in harmony with the planet. His story is a reminder that our food choices have far-reaching impacts on the environment and that by choosing plant-based options, we can contribute to a more sustainable and eco-friendly world.

This chapter has shed light on the environmental benefits of veganism, showing that it's not just a dietary choice, but a lifestyle choice that can significantly impact our planet's health. In the following chapters, we will delve deeper into the ethical considerations of veganism and explore how this lifestyle aligns with the principles of animal rights and compassion.

At the heart of veganism lies a deep ethical conviction about animal rights and welfare. This chapter explores the ethical underpinnings of veganism, looking at how the decision to avoid animal products is not only a personal health choice but also a stance against animal exploitation and cruelty. It delves into the philosophy of animal rights, understanding that every creature has an inherent value and the right to live free from suffering.

Consider the journey of Emma, an animal rights activist and documentary filmmaker from Melbourne. Emma's path to veganism began when she started working on a documentary about factory farming. Through her lens, she witnessed the realities of animal agriculture - the cramped conditions, the lack of freedom, and the ultimate fate of the animals. This experience profoundly impacted Emma, leading her to embrace veganism as a way to align her lifestyle with her values of compassion and non-violence.

Emma's veganism went beyond her diet. She became an advocate for animal rights, using her films to educate others about the conditions of animals in the agriculture industry. She highlighted not only the suffering of animals in factory farms but also the emotional and social complexity of these creatures. Her work shed light on the intelligence and sentience of animals, challenging the traditional view of animals as mere commodities.

Her activism extended to other areas of animal exploitation as well. Emma campaigned against the use of animals in entertainment, such as circuses and marine parks, where animals are often kept in unnatural and stressful conditions. She also advocated against animal testing, promoting cruelty-free and vegan products that do not rely on animal testing for their development.

One of Emma's key messages was about making ethical choices in everyday life. She encouraged people to think critically about where their food, clothing, and other products come from and to make choices that minimize harm to animals. She often shared her own experiences, discussing how she navigates challenges and stays true to her ethical principles.

Emma also explored the intersectionality of veganism with other social justice issues. She understood that the fight for animal rights is linked to broader struggles against exploitation and oppression. This perspective allowed her to connect with a wider audience and integrate her activism with other social causes.

Through her journey, Emma showed that veganism is more than a dietary choice; it's a commitment to a more ethical and just world. Her story illustrates that each decision we make can be a reflection of our values and an opportunity to stand against cruelty and exploitation.

This chapter has highlighted the ethical considerations and the importance of animal rights in veganism. It underscores the idea that veganism is a holistic approach to living, one that encompasses a deep respect and compassion for all living beings. In the next chapters, we will explore the community aspect of veganism, discussing how to find support, build networks, and engage in advocacy to promote a more compassionate and ethical world.

Veganism, at its core, is not just a personal journey; it's a movement built on shared values and community. This chapter explores the importance of community in the vegan lifestyle and the various ways vegans can engage in advocacy to promote understanding and acceptance of veganism. It highlights the power of collective action and support in making a more compassionate world.

Let's take a journey with Amina, a community organizer and vegan chef from Brooklyn, New York. Amina's vegan journey was initially a solitary one, but she soon realized the importance of community in sustaining and enriching her vegan lifestyle. She started by attending local vegan meetups, where she met like-minded individuals who shared her passion for plant-based living. These gatherings were more than social events; they were a source of inspiration, support, and collective wisdom.

Inspired by her new connections, Amina decided to use her skills as a chef to build community. She began hosting vegan cooking classes in her neighborhood, providing a space for people to learn about vegan cooking in a friendly, welcoming environment. These classes became about more than just food; they were a way for people to connect, share stories, and support each other in their vegan journeys. Amina also recognized the power of advocacy in promoting veganism. She organized community events to raise awareness about the benefits of a vegan lifestyle, not only for health but also for animal welfare and the environment. She partnered with local schools to introduce plant-based meals and provide nutrition education, helping to plant the seeds of change in the next generation.

Her advocacy extended to working with local businesses. Amina collaborated with restaurants and cafes in her area, encouraging them to add more vegan options to their menus. She provided them with recipes and insights into what vegans look for in dining out. This not only made vegan food more accessible in her community but also helped local businesses tap into a growing market.

Online, Amina created a digital platform for vegans in her area, a space where people could share resources, recipes, and tips. This virtual community became a vital source of support, especially for those who were new to veganism or lived in areas with few vegan-friendly options.

Amina's efforts showed that community and advocacy are integral to the vegan movement. Through her initiatives, she helped create a more inclusive and supportive environment for vegans and those curious about the lifestyle. Her story illustrates that everyone can play a role in building the vegan community, whether through organizing events, sharing knowledge, or simply being a supportive friend.

This chapter has underscored the importance of community and advocacy in veganism. It illustrates how building networks and engaging in collective action can not only support individual vegans but also promote broader societal acceptance and understanding of veganism. In the next chapters, we will explore the diverse global landscape of vegan cuisine, demonstrating how veganism is embraced and adapted in different cultures around the world.

Veganism, while a unified philosophy, manifests diversely across the globe, influenced by a variety of cultures, flavors, and culinary traditions. This chapter takes you on a gastronomic journey, exploring the rich tapestry of global vegan cuisine. It highlights how veganism adapts and thrives within different cultural contexts, offering a kaleidoscope of flavors, ingredients, and cooking techniques that enrich the vegan diet.

Let's travel with Ravi, a food blogger and avid traveler from London, who embarked on a journey to explore vegan cuisine around the world. Ravi's adventure began in India, a country known for its rich vegetarian tradition. Here, he discovered a plethora of vegan dishes steeped in history and flavor. Dishes like chana masala (spiced chickpeas), baingan bharta (smoked eggplant curry), and a variety of dal (lentil preparations) showcased how Indian cuisine naturally lends itself to veganism, using spices and herbs to create deeply flavorful dishes.

Moving east, Ravi explored the vegan scene in Japan. While traditional Japanese cuisine relies heavily on fish, Ravi found an array of vegan options influenced by Buddhist culinary practices. He savored dishes like miso soup made with seaweed instead of fish stock, inari sushi (sushi rice in a tofu pouch), and nasu dengaku (miso-glazed eggplant). He also discovered shojin ryori, a type of Japanese Buddhist cuisine that is entirely plant-based, focusing on seasonal ingredients and balance in flavors.

In the Middle East, Ravi was introduced to a variety of vegan-friendly dishes that are central to the region's culinary culture. Hummus, falafel, baba ganoush, tabbouleh, and stuffed vine leaves were not only delicious but also inherently vegan. He learned how these dishes are part of everyday eating in countries like Lebanon,

Israel, and Turkey, highlighting how vegan food can be both humble and celebratory. Ravi's journey then took him to Ethiopia, where he experienced the vegan-friendly tradition of fasting foods. During certain times of the year, many Ethiopians adhere to a vegan diet, abstaining from animal products. This practice has led to a rich variety of vegan dishes like injera (spongy flatbread) served with stews like misir wot (spicy lentils) and shiro (chickpea stew). The communal aspect of eating from a shared platter also underscored the social dimension of food in Ethiopian culture. In Mexico, Ravi delved into the vibrant flavors of Mexican cuisine, discovering vegan versions of traditional dishes. He enjoyed tacos filled with spicy grilled vegetables, black bean burritos, and guacamole with fresh tortillas. He also found that many traditional Mexican dishes are naturally vegan, such as salsas, rice, and beans, highlighting how vegan food is often ingrained in cultural culinary practices.

Through his travels, Ravi not only expanded his palate but also gained a deeper appreciation for the diversity of vegan cuisine. He learned that veganism is not a one-size-fits-all diet but a versatile and adaptable lifestyle that can be embraced in various cultural contexts.

This chapter has taken us on a culinary journey, showing the global diversity of vegan cuisine. It illustrates how veganism is not just a dietary choice but a cultural experience, offering a world of flavors, ingredients, and traditions to explore. In the following chapters, we will delve into the health benefits of a vegan diet, backed by scientific research, and address common myths and misconceptions about veganism.

The shift to a vegan lifestyle is often accompanied by a quest for better health and well-being. This chapter illuminates the myriad health benefits associated with veganism, supported by scientific research. It addresses how a well-planned vegan diet can contribute to improved health outcomes, including a lower risk of certain chronic diseases, better heart health, and enhanced overall wellness.

Let's explore the journey of Dr. Hannah Lee, a nutritionist and researcher from San Francisco, who has spent years studying the impacts of diet on health. Through her research, Dr. Lee has uncovered compelling evidence supporting the health benefits of a vegan diet.

One significant area of her research focuses on heart health. Studies have shown that a vegan diet, rich in fruits, vegetables, whole grains, nuts, and seeds, can improve heart health. This is largely due to the diet's lower levels of saturated fats, cholesterol, and higher levels of dietary fiber. Dr. Lee's research found that individuals following a vegan diet often have lower blood pressure and a reduced risk of heart disease compared to non-vegans.

Another area where Dr. Lee found vegan diets to be particularly beneficial is in the prevention and management of type 2 diabetes. A plant-based diet, low in fat and high in fiber, can improve insulin sensitivity and help regulate blood sugar levels. Her studies have shown that individuals on a vegan diet can have a significantly lower risk of developing type 2 diabetes and, in some cases, can even manage and reverse the condition.

Dr. Lee also explored the connection between diet and cancer prevention. Her research indicated that vegan diets might reduce the risk of certain types of cancer, particularly those related to the digestive system, like colorectal cancer. This protective effect is attributed to the high intake of fruits, vegetables, and legumes, which are rich in fiber, vitamins, and phytochemicals with cancer-protective properties.

Additionally, Dr. Lee's research touched on weight management. She found that people following a vegan diet tend to have a lower body mass index (BMI) compared to those on omnivorous diets. The natural tendency for vegan diets to be lower in calories and higher in dietary fiber helps with satiety and weight control, making it an effective lifestyle for those looking to manage their weight.

Beyond physical health, Dr. Lee's studies also looked at the mental health benefits of veganism. Emerging research suggests that the nutrients found in plant-based foods, such as antioxidants and phytochemicals, can have a positive impact on mental health. Some studies have indicated lower rates of depression and anxiety among those following a vegan diet.

Dr. Lee's journey and research highlight that a vegan diet, when well-planned and balanced, can offer substantial health benefits. However, she also emphasizes the importance of ensuring a sufficient intake of certain nutrients, such as vitamin B12, omega-3 fatty acids, iron, calcium, and vitamin D, which can be lower in a vegan diet. She advocates for a mindful approach to veganism, where individuals are not only conscious of eliminating animal products but also of nourishing their bodies with a diverse range of plant-based foods.

In this chapter, we have shed light on the health benefits and scientific research supporting veganism. It underscores the fact that veganism is not just a compassionate choice for animals and the environment, but also a beneficial one for personal health. In the next chapters, we will delve into practical tips and strategies for those looking to transition to a vegan lifestyle, ensuring a smooth and enjoyable journey.

The beauty of veganism lies in its versatility and adaptability across various culinary traditions around the world. This chapter takes you on a culinary exploration of veganism in global cuisines, showcasing the myriad of ways in which traditional dishes from different cultures can be enjoyed in a vegan context. It's a testament to the creativity and innovation that vegan cooking inspires, transcending boundaries and uniting us through the universal language of food.

Embark on this journey with Marco, a chef and food blogger from Rome, who has a passion for exploring vegan interpretations of classic dishes from around the globe. Marco's adventure begins in his home country, Italy, where he reinvents traditional Italian dishes with plant-based ingredients. His vegan lasagna, made with layers of cashew-based ricotta, spinach, and rich tomato sauce, is a hit among his followers, proving that Italian cuisine can be just as delicious without dairy or meat. Marco then takes his culinary exploration to Japan, a country known for its delicate flavors and fresh ingredients. He discovers the versatility of tofu and seaweed, staples in Japanese cuisine, which he uses to create vegan versions of sushi, miso soup, and tempura. He is particularly fascinated by the concept of umami, a flavor profile central to Japanese cooking, which he learns to achieve using ingredients like mushrooms and soy sauce.

Next, Marco ventures into the heart of India, where vegetarianism has deep cultural and religious roots. He is amazed by the diversity of dishes that are naturally vegan or can be easily adapted. He experiments with lentils, chickpeas, and an array of spices to create dishes like chana masala, aloo gobi, and dal. Marco finds that Indian cuisine's use of spices and herbs adds depth and richness to vegan dishes, making them incredibly flavorful and satisfying.

In Mexico, Marco explores the robust and vibrant flavors of Mexican cuisine. He discovers that many Mexican staples like beans, corn, and avocados are vegan-friendly. He experiments with making vegan tacos, using jackfruit as a substitute for meat, and creates rich, spicy salsas to accompany them. He also learns to make tamales with vegan fillings, a dish that proves to be a fun challenge and a hit with his audience.

Marco's journey also takes him to the Middle East, where he explores the rich flavors of Lebanese, Israeli, and Persian cuisines. He finds a plethora of vegan options in dishes like hummus, baba ganoush, falafel, and tabbouleh. He is inspired by the use of legumes, nuts, and fresh herbs, which are central to many dishes in the region.

Through his travels and culinary experiments, Marco not only broadens his cooking repertoire but also shares his experiences with his followers, inspiring them to explore the diversity of vegan cuisine. His journey illustrates that veganism can be a delicious, creative, and culturally enriching experience.

In this chapter, we have traveled with Marco through various cuisines around the world, discovering the rich diversity of vegan cooking. It shows that embracing a vegan lifestyle does not mean giving up the flavors and dishes one loves but rather rediscovering them in a new, compassionate, and sustainable way. In the next chapter, we will conclude this guide with a reflection on the journey of veganism, offering insights and inspirations for continuing this rewarding and impactful path.

As we reach the conclusion of this guide, it's a time for reflection and forward-thinking. Embracing veganism is not just about adopting a new diet; it's about embarking on a lifelong journey of discovery, growth, and alignment with one's values of compassion, health, and sustainability. This final chapter is dedicated to summing up the essence of the vegan journey and offering guidance on how to continue this fulfilling and impactful path.

Consider the story of Julia, a teacher and mother from Vancouver, who embarked on her vegan journey two years ago. Initially motivated by health reasons, Julia's understanding and practice of veganism deepened over time, becoming an integral part of her identity. She found joy in cooking plant-based meals for her family, exploring new ingredients and recipes, and was delighted to see her children develop a taste for a variety of fruits, vegetables, and grains.

Julia also experienced challenges, particularly in social settings where vegan options were limited. But these challenges became opportunities for advocacy and education. She found gentle and effective ways to share her choices with others, leading by example and often dispelling myths about veganism through her own healthy and vibrant lifestyle.

As Julia continued on her journey, she learned the importance of community. Joining local vegan groups and online forums, she found support, shared experiences, and made new friendships. These connections provided her with the encouragement and resources she needed to maintain her commitment to veganism.

Julia also discovered the broader implications of her lifestyle choices. She became more conscious of her impact on the environment, opting for sustainable and ethical products beyond her diet. She engaged in local initiatives for animal rights and environmental conservation, finding fulfillment in contributing to causes that resonated with her values.

One of the most significant aspects of Julia's journey was the continuous learning and personal growth. She kept herself informed about the latest research on vegan nutrition, ensuring that her diet remained balanced and healthy. She also explored the philosophical and ethical dimensions of veganism, which deepened her commitment and understanding of the lifestyle.

As Julia's story illustrates, the vegan journey is unique for each individual. It's a path of exploration, learning, and adaptation. It's about making choices that align with one's values and finding joy and fulfillment in those choices.

To continue your vegan journey, remember the importance of staying informed, connected, and open to learning. Keep exploring new foods, recipes, and cuisines. Engage with the vegan community, either locally or online, and consider how you can contribute to advocacy and education efforts. Stay abreast of the latest research in vegan nutrition to ensure your diet remains healthy and balanced.

Most importantly, be compassionate with yourself. Understand that veganism is a journey and that perfection is not the goal. It's about making conscious choices that align with your values and doing the best you can at any given moment.

As we close this guide, remember that your vegan journey is a powerful statement of your commitment to a healthier, more ethical, and sustainable world. It's a journey that can bring immense personal fulfillment and a positive impact on the world around you. Keep exploring, learning, and growing on your path, and know that you are part of a global community of individuals dedicated to making a difference.